HAWAIIAN DIET

Hawaiian Vegetables and Their Function in the Diet

Kyle P. Rutter

Table of Contents

CHAPTER 1

VERY SIMPLE HAWAIIAN RECIPES

These Hawaiian recipes will truly completely motive you to experience such as you live in heaven with their grand heady fragrance and choice!

Hawaii is widely known for its sandy coasts and abundant develop. However have fact be instructed you tried actual Hawaiian meals?

On the off hazard that factor of reality, I`m precise that at last, you can not cease considering it. Or some thing awful may happen, after which that is your possibility to stumble upon the islands' combo of dispositions.

Specific, you would possibly conceivably procure Hawaiian pizza anyplace, but there is some other facet to Hawaiian meals whilst contrasted with that.

From kalua red meat to mai tais, those recipes will definitely completely fulfill your inclination.

These 26 general recipes will simply completely deliver

the neighborhood choice of Hawaii into your home!

Hawaii is well-known for its sandy coasts and abundant develop. However have as a count number of reality you tried valid Hawaiian meals?

Want to shop this recipe? Go into your e mail under and we're going to ship the recipe directly for an inbox!

Hawaiian Chicken with Smoked Pineapple

In the occasion that undoubtedly, I'm precise that at last, you cannot cease considering it. Or the outcomes can be severe, then, at that factor that is your possibility to stumble upon the islands' combo of dispositions.

Specific, you would possibly doubtlessly advantage Hawaiian pizza anyplace, but there is some other facet to Hawaiian meals whilst contrasted with that.

From kalua red meat to mai tais, those recipes will truly completely fulfill your inclination.

These 26 general recipes will simply completely deliver

the neighborhood choice of Hawaii into your home!

Hawaiian Pizza - Sally's Food association Dependence

Sally's Food association Dependence.

CHAPTER 2

HAWAIIAN PIZZA

Hawaiian pizza could be much counseled globally. While a few won't love this pizza inclination, I loads of maximum surely am!

It has absolutely terrific, appalling, and stinky dispositions in a unmarried attack.

Goodness, I'm denying through and through. Assuming which you are additionally, here is a totally simple recipe for residence made Hawaiian pizza.

This recipe, regularly, needs for residence made pizza mixture. However it is a snap to develop, and you may truly simply want 6 general components.

The final results should be a thick, delectable overlaying that could possibly maintain the sauce, cheddar, red meat things, pineapple things, and bacon nibbled small amounts. Yum!

Hawaiian Chicken

Supper on the Zoo

Hawaiian Chicken Recipe | Smoked Chicken | Pineapple Chicken #hen #grilling #dinner #pineapple #dinneratthezoo

2. Hawaiian Chicken

These hen thighs are marinated in a coconut milk mix, then smoked to quality.

Use with succulent pineapple things, and you may truly get a tropical-pro hen supper!

The pivotal to such amazing dispositions is getting the marinade ideal. Try now no longer to concern; it is very smooth to deliver.

Want to shop this recipe? Go into your e mail under and we're going to ship the recipe directly for an inbox!

You will simply honestly require earthy coloured sugar, sesame oil, garlic, soy sauce, and coconut milk.

You may doubtlessly make use of this hen dish over a mattress of white rice. In the occasion that you are feeling beneficent, installation the rice in coconut milk for covered dispositions!

Three. Fricke Deal with Mix

This counseled Hawaiian association with includes terrific and stinky dispositions, putting off a habit-forming dish you would possibly find to everybody.

On the off hazard which you're now no longer taught with reference to furikake, it is an simply completely dry flavoring comprising of toasted sesame seeds, inexperienced growth, sugar, and salt.

With three bins of grains and chips of your choice, you would possibly doubtlessly make a large lay out of this association with combo.

The furikake enters the margarine soy sauce syrup, growing wonderful inclination mixes.

Hawaiian Deep-broiled Rice

Life within side the Loft residence.

CHAPTER 3

HAWAIIAN DEEP-BROILED RICE

Incredibly trustworthy Hawaiian snacks functionality this flavor-pressed pan fried rice. It has absolutely all that paperwork the first rate Hawaiian choice – red meat, chime pepper, and typically, pineapples.

Fabricating this dish is an first-rate manner to cope with makes use of your intending to be rice. Use it for entertaining, and the web website online visitors will simply now no longer droop which you made make use of bloodless day-antique rice. The loosening up dispositions, the fleecy look — it is critically amazing!

Hawaiian Chicken Kebabs (with Pineapple!) - Cooking Elegant

Cooking Elegant

5. Hawaiian Chicken Kebabs

These smoked Hawaiian enjoyments consolidate marinated hen, pineapples, crimson onions, and ringer peppers. The final results is one of the maximum stable hen kebabs previously!

I critically love hen recipes, and I fee kebabs. So doubtlessly, that is a victory for me. Make it on your island-propelled summer time length party, and I'm precise it is going to be a struck.

This dish makes use of kitchen place staples, but you may simply procure a elegant inclination and sensitive strikes.

There aren't any awesome components or highly-priced devices required. Perk, the cooking time is simply 15 mins!

6. Hawaiian Macaroni Salad

Commonplace, very simple, and pretty velvety, this macaroni salad will simply completely swipe the find at out of doors BBQ occasions or possibly in first rate stop of the week ruin damage recipes.

Assuming which you're surely to post to the conventional recipe for this facet dish, you may simply basically require carrots, organized macaroni, salt, pepper, and mayonnaise. Throw the entirety with every one-of-a-kind other, that's it!

The serving of blended veggies is a touch crucial at the mayo, but this is the important to the easy look.

For a valid and changed and settled rendition, you would possibly doubtlessly alternative the mayo with Greek yogurt or veggie lover mayo.

Sluggish Cooker Braised Hawaiian Pineapple Chicken Tacos.

Insane Collect

Sluggish Cooker Braised Hawaiian Pineapple Chicken Tacos | halfbakedharvest.com

CHAPTER 4

HAWAIIAN PINEAPPLE CHICKEN TACOS

Anticipate a mix of dispositions from those stacked sassy tacos! Delicate hen with hula sauce, a reasonably heat slaw, and crunchy Eastern noodles heaps those madly amazing tacos.

For the sauce, you may simply require garlic, soy sauce, hundreds of pineapple juice, pineapple things, honey, and ginger. This is going with the hen, withinside the slow cooker.

There's an extra motion of searing, but it is so nicely absolutely justified! This yields caramelized destroyed hen with instead clean sides.

Pork and Cheese Sliders

Enjoy With Dimes

We maximum surely fee those cushy red meat and cheddar sliders. They are a especially exceptional lunch or tidbit!

8. Pork and Cheese Sliders

Ideal for a noontime control or a mild supper recipe, those sliders consolidate common components: red meat and cheddar.

CHAPTER 5

HAWAIIAN OAT DISH

BEGIN YOUR DAY BECOMING WITH THIS BENEFICENT AND SOUND AND ALTERED AND SETTLED OAT DISH. THIS MORNING MEAL DISH IS CHOCK STACKED WITH SUPER DISPOSITIONS AND HAS VIRTUALLY A NOTEWORTHY SYSTEM.

THE REDUCE ALMONDS AND TOASTED DESTROYED COCONUT WILL EASILY ABSOLUTELY REVEL IN YOUR FEEL OF FLAVOR AT EVERY ATTACK. ALSO, WITHOUT A DOUBT, THIS OAT DISH WILL

UNDOUBTEDLY NOW NO LONGER BE "HAWAIIAN" WITH OUT THE PINEAPPLE GOODIES!

13. hawaiian coleslaw

ASSUMING YOU`RE GETTING BORED WITH WELL-KNOWN SLAW, THIS RECIPE BRINGS A NOVEL, NEW ASPECT TO THE TABLE.

CAUTIOUSLY FANTASTIC WITH SIMPLY THE PROPER QUANTITY OF PIECE ISSUE, THIS HAWAIIAN SERVING OF COMBINED VEGGIES IS A NOTABLE LAY OUT WITH SMOKED MEATS, POSITIONED INNER A TOASTED BUN.

IT PACKS A CITRUSY INCLINATION; LIKEWISE, A TON OF

AN ABUNDANCE OF WAY TO THE FRENCH DRESSING CLOTHING, MANGO STRONG SHAPES, AND PINEAPPLE NIBBLED SMALL AMOUNTS. USE IT AT YOUR OVERDUE SPRING SEASON LENGTH LUAU TO GROWTH THE THRILLING PUTTING!

14. fervor fruit bars

AMONG HAWAII'S PLENTY OF ADVISED DISPOSITIONS ORIGINATES FROM STRENGTH HERBAL PRODUCT. THIS YELLOW NATURAL PRODUCT, FURTHERMORE PORTRAYED AS LILIKOI, IS LARGELY AMONGST CERTAINLY CONSIDERED ONE AMONG POSSIBLY OF THE

MAXIMUM AMPLE THRILLING HERBAL PRODUCT AT THE ISLANDS.

PUREE THE LILIKOI, AND MIX IT IN WITH EGGS, SUGAR, AND FLOUR. PLAN TO QUALITY, AND YOU'LL EASILY STEADY YUMMY NATURAL PRODUCT BARS EMPOWERING YOU OF RAINBOWS AND DAYLIGHT.

SLUGGISH COOKER KALUA PORK - EASY, JUST THREE ENERGETIC PARTS! -

SKINNYTASTE

15. kalua pork

KALUA BEEF IS AN EXEMPLARY HAWAIIAN DISH THAT YOU MAY REGULARLY SONG DOWN

IN LUAUS. IT'S SMOKED DESTROYED BEEF NORMALLY ORGANIZED IN AN "IMU," OR RECORDED SUBTERRANEAN COOKTOP.

FORTUNATELY, WITH THIS RECIPE, YOU MIGHT NOT INCLUDE THE RELENTLESS REMEDY OF COOKING KALUA BEEF.

ALL YOU MAY REQUIRE IS A SLOWER COOKER IN AN EFFORT TO DO THE HUGE MAJORITY OF THE MANUAL YOU! UTILIZING REALLY THREE FIERY PARTS, YOU MAY HAVE A WET, DELICATE, AND SPECTACULAR SUPER SMOKY BEEF DISH FOR ENTERTAINING.

16. spam deep-broiled rice

HAWAIIANS LIKE SPAM A TON, SO IT IS SOMETHING HOWEVER A SURPRISE THAT THIS REPRESENT CONSUMES PLENTY OF JARS OF SPAM EACH YEAR.

IF YOU WANT THIS TINNED ELEGANT THIS SPAM PAN FRIED RICE IS A MUST-ATTEMPT. IT YIELDS A RECIPE OF SCRUMPTIOUS PAN FRIED RICE WITH A FIRST RATE SHAPE FROM CONSOLIDATED VEGGIES.

full it off with sriracha sauce for a heat kick!

hawaiian shoyu chicken

SUPPER, SOMETIME LATER DEAL WITH

17. shoyu chicken

ONE GREATER DISH THAT MAKES USE OF A TERRIFI INCLINATION BLEND IS SHOYU FOWL, A DISH WITH BEGINNING FACTORS FROM JAPAN.

AMONG ITS FOUNDATIONS, SHOYU, IS JAPANESE-FASHION SOY SAUCE THIS IS AMPLE IN UMAMI DISPOSITIONS.

THE SOY SAUCE ENTERS WITHINSIDE THE MARINADE ALONG DIVERSE DISTINCT PREFERENCES. BLEND ANYTHING IN WITH THE FOWL AND KEEP IT WITHINSIDE THE FRIDGE OVERNIGHT.

YOU CAN FISH FRY THE MARINATED FOWL FOR AN EXEMPLARY BBQ INCLINATION OR SET IT UP WITHINSIDE THE COOKTOP TO PROVIDE A SUCCULENT AND SHABBY FOWL DISH.

18. hawaiian fruit salad

THIS HERBAL PRODUCT SALAD IS LARGELY MOST OF THE MAXIMUM APPEALING PREPARATIONS WITH I ACTUALLY HAVE EARLIER THAN HAD IN FACT. DYNAMIC WITH CONSOLIDATED INGREDIENTS GROWN FROM THE FLOOR IN A PINEAPPLE BOAT, IT IS A ACTUAL EYE-CATCHER AND INSTITUTION PLEASER!

ASSUMING YOU WANT CERTAINLY CONSIDERED ONE AMONG A TYPE, SCRUMPTIOUS NATURAL PRODUCTS, YOU MAY DISCOVER THEM RIGHT RECORDED BELOW ON THIS PLATE OF COMBINED VEGGIES.

PINEAPPLES, ORANGES, STRAWBERRIES, AND INEXPERIENCED GRAPES ARE UNDENIABLY CONSOLIDATED IN A HEAVENLY, YOGURT-PRIMARILY BASED TOTALLY CLOTHING.

PASSIONFRUIT CURD DOUGHNUTS

HUMMINGBIRD HIGH

19. passionfruit donuts

THESE SPARKLING DOUGHNUTS ARE OVERFLOWING WITH FLAVORFUL STRENGTH HERBAL PRODUCT CURD, AND THOSE BREADS WILL CARRY AN UNMISTAKABLY MOMENTOUS CHOICE FOR A TABLE.

SAFEGUARDED WITH POWDERED SUGAR, THOSE MODEST SEARCHING DOUGHNUTS ARE VERY MILD AND DEFROST VALID FOR YOUR MOUTH.

VARIOUS DISTINCT VARIATIONS OF THIS RECIPE MAKE USE OF COCONUT OR PINEAPPLES FOR THE ORAL DENTAL FILLING.

CHAPTER 6

HAWAIIAN ROLLS

HAWAIIAN ROLLS ARE A BIT WONDERFUL, CUSHIONED, MILD, AND CRUNCHY. THEY'RE TYPICALLY SOMETHING THAT APPEAL FOR YOU IN RESIDENCE MADE ROLLS.

THE PINEAPPLE JUICE BRINGS THE HAWAIIAN INCLINATION, EVEN AS THE HONEY LIFTS THE OVERALL FIRST-RATE INCLINATION.

YOU CAN CONSUME THOSE ROLLS CLEAR, BUT THEY MAY BE

HIGHER WHILE SLATHERED WITH HONEY MARGARINE!

21. hawaiian rice treat

THIS RICE DEAL WITH IS IMPARTED WITH DISPOSITIONS OF CREAM CHEDDAR, PINEAPPLE, AND VANILLA. IT'S OBVIOUSLY MY ADVISED HAWAIIAN BENEFIT FOOD.

THE BLEND OF PINEAPPLE SAUCE AND HEAVENLY CHEDDAR COULD BE VERY FLAVORFUL.

PERK, YOU MAY GET AN AMPLE DEAL WITH THAT ISN'T ALWAYS PRECISELY CERTAINLY EXCESSIVELY SURPRISING. EAT IT AGREEABLE OR COLD;

REGARDLESS, YOU MAY STAY IN FOR AN BENEFIT!

BLUE HAWAIIAN RECIPE

FOOD MAKING PLANS CHARM

22. blue hawaiian

2 OF AMONGST ONE OF THE MAXIMUM ADVISED HAWAIIAN NATURAL PRODUCT DISPOSITIONS LIVE ON THIS LIQUOR CONSUME: PINEAPPLE AND COCONUT.

buy

ORCHESTRATE PROGRAMS WITHINSIDE THE HAZINESS

AWS OFFERS FINANCIALLY SAVVY METHODS TO ADDRESS PREPARE AND ASSEMBLE WEBWEB SITES AND INTERNET PROGRAMS,

MAKING USE OF ANY FORM OF FORM OF CMS.

PLAN TO CERTAINLY ABSOLUTELY SENSE THE OVERDUE SPRING SEASON LENGTH PUTTING THE MIN YOU ARE TAKING A FLAVOR!

THIS SUMMERY CONSUME ESSENTIALLY CALLS FOR THREE VIVACIOUS PARTS — COCONUT RUM, PINEAPPLE SQUEEZE, AND BLUE CURACAO.

THE ULTIMATE ENTHUSIASTIC DYNAMIC SOLVING RESOURCES THE CONSUME A BLUE TONE, SEARCHING JUST LIKE THE

CERTAINLY CONSIDERED ONE AMONG A TYPE WATERS.

A BLUE HAWAIIAN MAY BE GIVEN FROSTY OR AT THE ROCKS. WHICHEVER YOU PICK, IT'S GOING TO SHIELD YOU REVIVED AT THE CUSHTY DAYS.

23. mai tai

THE MAI TAI IS RIGHT LIQUOR IN TIKI CULTURE. EXTRAORDINARY PREPARATIONS OF SEE THIS LIQUOR AS A STUPID CONSUME DUE TO ITS DYNAMIC TONE, BUT IT DOES PARCELS A LIQUOR STRIKE.

THIS CONSUME INCLUDES DIM AND EARTHY YELLOW RUM AS

A BASE, WITH PROTECTED DISPOSITIONS FROM SQUEEZED ORANGE AND LIME JUICE.

BLEND ANYTHING IN A LIQUOR SHAKER, AND YOU'LL HAVE AN EXEMPLARY EXTRAORDINARY CONSUME IN MINS.

WHITE TASTY HEAVENLY CHOCOLATE CHIP COOKIES

24. white tasty heavenly chocolate macadamia nut cookies

MACADAMIA NUTS ARE A AREA PRIZE IN HAWAII, SO PEOPLE THERE ABSOLUTELY REALIZE ABSOLUTELY THE EXCELLENT

METHOD TO CONSUME THEM THE PROPER STRATEGY!

SOME WANT THEM DIRECT, EVEN AS OTHERS LIKE FLAVORED OR CHOCOLATEY NUTS.

AS A WAYS AS I IS PROBABLY CONCERNED, I WANT THOSE NUTS IN CRUNCHY, AGREEABLE TREATS! HOWEVER THAT ISN'T ALL CONSIDERING THE FACT THAT THOSE TREATS ADDITIONALLY HAVE WHITE DELECTABLE PLEASANT CHOCOLATE CHIPS.

TAKE DISPLAY THE STICKING TO EVEN OUT THROUGH MAKING USE OF SIMMERED NUTS IN PLACE OF CRUDE ONES.

I ASSURE THAT THE PROTECTED MOVEMENT OF BROILING IS CERTIFIED FOR IT FOR THAT REASON OF THE AMPLIFIED INCLINATION AND FRAGRANCE.

SUPPORTIVE OF TIP: CONSIST OF GREATER BROWN CONTRASTED WITH WHITE SUGAR WITH THIS DEAL WITH COMBINATION TO

Direct Dough for Bread Newbie's

This is a extraordinarily truthful batter recipe for novices. You actually need clearly 6 vital vivacious parts, perk a tad cornmeal for putting in place the fry dish. (You can byskip up that every time required.) A lot of the instant is fingers off because the batter scales. You should ponder... why shed the instant while you could simply collect frigid pizza batter? Frosty pizza combination is maximum genuinely difficulty free, but with none training masking has first rate inclination and appearance that basically originates from new batter. What`s extra, you could make use of the batter for cheddar breadsticks, as nicely!

Guests Andy remarked: "Incredibly direct, very speedily, exceedingly eminent! I should do with out raw thick pizzas and

I discover with this recipe that I could make them skinny and crunchy; I like essentially precisely the manner wherein clean it is. I make pizza 1 or 2 instances every month! Have now no longer gotten one for alternatively time as of now! ★★★★★"

In the occasion which you have totally made unbiased bagels or sandwich bread, you could serenely make pizza combination because it is speedier, a high-quality deal substantially much less made complex, and requirements significantly much less sporting events.

Independent pizza on meals readiness sheet

Recap: Self-made Pizza Dough Energetic parts

All pizza combination starts offevolved with the indistinguishable vital enthusiastic parts: flour, yeast, splash, salt, and olive oil. Here is the damage down of what I make use of in my unbiased pizza outdoor recipe. The complete printable recipe is here.

Yeast: I make use of Platinum Yeast from Red Celeb.

I even have without a doubt the great very last merchandise after I make use of this short yeast. The Platinum yeast is notable because its cognizant equation helps your batter and makes fabricating cooperating with yeast vital. You essentially want 1 normal association of yeast (2 and 1/four teaspoons) to complete the paintings.

Splash: I analyzed this pizza batter recipe with numerous measures of shower. 1 and 1/three cups is the notable sum. Utilize agreeable splash to dwindled ascent time, stressing

100-110°F. Anything over 130°F disposes of the yeast.

Flour: Make usage of unbleached average spherical white flour on this recipe. Easing up the flour strips away numerous of the sound and changed strong protein, in order to have an effect on basically what does it intervene with you? Shower the flour ingests. You should selection bread at any factor flour for a chewier pizza hull. Assuming you want complete grain bread, strive this complete wheat pizza combination all matters being equal.

Oil: A set Tablespoons of delivered virgin olive oil contains of awesome inclination to the combination. Try now no longer to forget about to make certain to comb the combination with olive oil within side the beyond comprising of the garnishes, which receives as opposed to the outdoor layer from analyzing soaked.

Salt: Salt contains of required inclination.

Sugar: 1 Tbsp of sugar builds the yeast's profession in addition to soften the combination, explicitly while matched with truly olive oil.

Cornmeal: Cornmeal isn't always precisely absolutely within side the batter, but it is applied to tidy the pizza fry skillet. Cornmeal substances the pizza outdoor truly delivered inclination in addition to fresh. The extra a part of conveyance pizzas you esteem have sincerely cornmeal below hull!

You would possibly possibly correspondingly include of one tsp each garlic powder in addition to Italian flavoring blend to the batter while you include of the flour. Guests Shane remarked: "Exceptional pizza batter. I include of stressing 1 tabs of garlic powder in addition to Italian all-normal ordinary spices to provide the batter extra inclination along forty grams of cornmeal for a spell circumstance. It freezes nicely in addition to makes a putting skinny hull. ★★★★★"

2 pics of unbiased pizza batter in a ball in addition to scaling in a pitcher recipe on reply to

This is a Lean Bread Dough

Pizza outdoor layer, just like unbiased bagels, craftsman's bread, in addition to focaccia, requests a lean combination. A lean combination does not make use of eggs or margarine. Without the extra fats introduction the combination delicate, you are assured a dry pizza masking. (In any case, I assist making use of a few olive oil for inclination in addition to to usually hold up with the interior at the gentler side.) Recipes like supper rolls in addition to in a single day cinnamon rolls request fats to create a "considerable combination," which produces a milder in addition to extra pastry like bread.

Pizza Dough with Toppings withinside the Previous Food readiness

Recap: Methods to Make Easy Pizza Dough

Make the batter: Mix the combination energetic dynamic fixings with every distinct different the difficult manner or make use of a hand held or stand blender. Do this in sporting events as decided within side the created recipe recorded here.

Ply: Knead manually or misfortune the batter together along with your blender. I like doing this via way of means of hand additionally as you could genuinely fee me within side the video cut.

Rise:

Area

Combination right into a lubed mixing recipe, cowls solidly, in addition to dispense to ascend for stressing ninety minutes or in a single day within side the cooler.

Strike and make: Strike down climbed combination to supply air bubbles. Partition in 2. Carry combination out right into a 12-inch circle. Cover in addition to relaxation as you prep paintings the pizza garnishes.

Top it: Top with willing closer to pizza fixings.

Plan: Prepare pizza at an truly warm temperature for basically stressing 15 minutes.

Youthful chefs can genuinely assist AND having a high-quality time on the identical time. Empower the younger human beings help you with assessing down the combination in addition to make right into a circle. They can genuinely include in their cheeses in addition to make pepperoni encounters along the pie. That should do without a smiley pizza?

Inclined closer to Pizza Frying broiling dish

Empower me percentage my pinnacle choices for pizza searing broiling box simply in state of affairs you are getting every other one. I make use of in addition to like (subsidiary internet connects) this lay out in addition to this lay out. On the off danger which you like meals making plans your unbiased pizzas on pizza rocks, I even have absolutely applied this embedded within side the beyond in addition to it is perfect.

In the occasion which you do not have without a doubt a pizza fry box, make use of a ordinary sheet fry skillet. Oil it with olive oil in addition to

Area

The aggregate ball(s) into man or woman zipped-pinnacle bag(s) in addition to blanketed solidly, pushing out all of the air. Ice for as much as ninety days.

FAQ: Simply precisely how Do I Thaw Icy Pizza Dough?

Area

The frigid pizza aggregates within side the cooler for stressing eight hrs or overnight. At the factor whilst organized introduction pizza, dispose of the batter from the refrigerator in addition to make it viable for to relaxation for thirty mins at the reply to. Wage motion five within side the recipe recorded here.

Simple House made Pizza Dough

Recipe pile up star Recipe four. Nine from 588 investigates

Creator:

- Sally
- Prep paintings Time:
- 2 hrs, 15 minutes

- Get equipped Time:
- 15 minutes
- Full Time:
- 2 hrs, 50% a hr
- Create:
- 2 12-inch pizzas
- PIN RECIPE
- Remarks
- PRINT the RECIPE

Recap

Follow those vital hints for a thick, fresh, in addition to crunchy pizza out of doors layer on your domestic. The recipe yields enough pizza aggregate for two 12-inch pizzas additionally as you could clearly ice up part of the batter for a few different time. Near 2 greater extra kilos of aggregate full.

Fiery dynamic fixings

1 in addition to 1/three cups (320ml) snug shower (among 100-110°F, 38-43°C)

2 in addition to 1/four teaspoons (7g) Platinum Yeast from Red Celeb rapid yeast (1 everyday packet)*

1 Tbsp (13g) granulated sugar

2 Tablespoons (30ml) olive oil, motivator something else for fry skillet in addition to purging on batter

1 tsp salt

Three in addition to 1/2 cups (stressing 450g) all-spherical flour (spoon and evened out), motivation something else for fingers in addition to floor area splash of cornmeal for purifying the fry dish

Directions

Blend the snug splash, yeast, in addition to granulated sugar with every one-of-a-kind different within side the recipe of your stand blender geared up with a batter snare or oar gadget. Cover in addition to make it viable for to relaxation for five minutes. *If you don`t have without a doubt a stand blender, basically make use of a massive mixing recipe in addition to mixture the batter in with a wooden spoon or elastic spatula within side the sticking to action.

Comprise of the olive oil, salt, in addition to flour. Misfortune on delivered down fee for two minutes. Change the batter out right into a lightly floured floor area.

. With cautiously floured fingers, ply the aggregate for three-four minutes (for a visual, admire me do it within side the video reduce over!). The batter can clearly be a bit moreover massive for a blender to paintings it, anyhow you could clearly really make use of the blender on delivered down fee all matters being equal. Subsequent to plying, the aggregate should really nonetheless really truly sense a bit delicate. Hit it together along with your finger - within side the occasion that it constantly jumps back, your batter receives equipped to rise. Or something horrific would possibly happen, hold to massage.

Carefully oil a vital dinner with oil or nonstick splash absolutely make use of the specific same banquet you applied for the batter.

Area the aggregate within side the banquet, reworking it to layer all aspects within side the oil. Cover the banquet with light-weight mild weight aluminum foil, plastic cowl, or spotless meals making plans area

Towel. Permit the batter to climb at area temperature degree diploma for 60-ninety minutes or up until dual in estimation. (Thought: For the snug laying out on an mainly famous day, snug your range to 150°F (66°C). Change the broiler off, area the aggregate inner, and preserve the entryway incredibly barely open. This may be a satisfied with laying out on your batter to rise. In the wake of stressing 50% a hr, close the range entryway to capture the air inner with the supporting aggregate. At the factor whilst it is upgraded in estimation, put off from the range.)

Preheat range to 475°F (246°C). Permit it to snug for a trifling of 15-20 minutes as you're making the pizza. (In the occasion that using a pizza shake, area

it within side the broiler to preheat moreover.) Delicately oil meals making plans sheet or pizza fry skillet with nonstick splash or olive oil. Shower cautiously with cornmeal, which offers the out of doors extra problem and inclination.

Make the aggregate: When the batter receives equipped, strike it to offer any sort of sort of air bubbles. Partition the batter down the middle. (Or, greater than probably assembling 2 pizzas, ice up part of the batter for a few different time. See crisp guidelines beneath.) On a cautiously floured run floor area using lightly floured fingers or shifting pin, absolutely squash the batter right into a circle. Position on pre-organized fry field and, using cautiously floured fingers, put off and squash the plate right into a 12-inch circle, stressing 1/2-inch thick. On the off danger that the batter jelly decreasing as you goal to attract out it, live farfar from what you are doing, cowl it cautiously for five-10 minutes, then, at that factor, try as soon as greater.

When fashioned right into a 12-inch circle, increment the aspect of the aggregate round lay out a lip regarding the perimeters. I basically capture the perimeters round lay out the aspect. On the off danger that using a pizza shake, area the aggregate proper on pastry specialist's strips off tidied up with cornmeal.

Cover batter cautiously with plastic cowl or spotless meals making plans area towel and allow to relaxation for numerous minutes as you installation your pizza fixings. I advise pepperoni and inexperienced peppers or jalapeño matters, extra cheddar pizza, Hawaiian pizza, marguerite pizza, pesto pizza, spinach artichoke white pizza, or domestic made BBQ chicken pizza.

Top and installation the pizza: Making usage of your fingers, force troubles into the floor area of the aggregate to keep away from murmuring. To keep away from the oral dental filling from assembling your pizza overlaying soaked, easy the pinnacle cautiously with olive oil. Top together along with your desired fixings and plan for 13-

15 minutes or up until the hull is gold brown.

Thing snug pizza and use quickly. Cover intending to be pizza emphatically and preserve up with within side the refrigerator. Warm as you pick. Prepared pizza matters can clearly be frigid near ninety days.

THE END

www.ingramcontent.com/pod-product-compliance
Lightning Source LLC
LaVergne TN
LVHW010120170826
845678LV00012B/2513

* 9 7 9 8 3 6 7 3 9 2 1 6 6 *